Also by Jacquelyn Small
TRANSFORMERS: The Therapists of the Future

BECOMING
NATURALLY
THERAPEUTIC

JACQUELYN SMALL

REVISED EDITION

The Eupsychian Press
950 Roadrunner Road
Austin, Texas 78746

Library of Congress
Catalog Card Number: 81-65537   *1 - 89*

ISBN: 0-939344-00-9

Cover design and graphics: Bear Creek Studios, Austin, Texas 78737
Illustrations, page design: Rolf Tom Michelsen, Awareness Art Graphics, Brookhaven, N.Y.

Printing History: July 1981 B5, November 1983 A5, May 1985 B25, October 1985 B25, July 1986 B5, July 1987 B5, April 1988 B5.

Published by:
The Eupsychian Press
950 Roadrunner Road
Austin, Texas 78746

Order From:
The Eupsychian Press
P.O. Box 3090
Austin, Texas 78764

Bookstore

BECOMING NATURALLY THERAPEUTIC

CONTENTS

Preface

In 1975 *Becoming Naturally Therapeutic* began circulating within the alcoholism treatment community as a little guidebook for alcoholism counselors seeking ways to become more confident and professional in their work with alcoholic clients. It achieved instant popularity, and I was rather amazed. To me, it was so simple and easy to write, I couldn't imagine why it was making such an impact. Since then, in receiving feedback from many who've read it, I've discovered the answer: *Becoming Naturally Therapeutic*—without explicitly saying so—is based on the universal Law of Love. And this law is totally transforming, for it is the force behind the essence of human purpose we are all designed to manifest in the world of relationship. *Everything* is relationship. And the Law of Love is what holds it all together!

Love is Truth. When Truth happens between two people, there is a *noticeable* exchange of energy. And conversely, when untruth prevails, no energy is exchanged—*nothing happens.* Therefore, untruth does not even exist. Love is Truth, and Truth is Reality.

In other words, the human personality is an instrument designed specifically to concretize the Law of Love in the world. And this universal law can only operate within the context of relationship—otherwise it remains an abstract, formless concept—nonexistent. If you will notice from your own experience, it is only through touching one another (and not just physically) and observing what we reflect for each other . . . what we learn . . . that we are able to know ourselves. We *re*mind each other of who we are. This is our purpose.

Becoming Naturally Therapeutic is a study of the human qualities inherent within the personality structure that manifest practically and simply the Law of Love. As you go through the book, studying and practicing the personality traits that are offered as ways to use oneself in a relationship, you will see they all bring about the absolute Truth of a situation—pointing the person to himself, honestly, simply.

Therapeutic relationship is no accident, nor is it a game: it is following the natural laws of human nature, bringing us closer and closer to the authenticity of our being. Toxic relationship is its opposite: taking us further and further away from who we are, fostering untruth.

Therapeutic relating can be recognized in operation, defined, taught, practiced and mastered. It is no mystery! It is Truth happening through a magnetic exchange of energy that makes dynamic contact with another, heals, and then transforms. This little book shows what it looks like in the here and now, day-to-day life of a person placed in the role of helper to one in trouble—as we all are from time to time.

Because of its universal application for all of us, we have now expanded this book, adding a chapter on Warmth (which research was not available when the first edition was written), and including the genius of our illustrator, Rolf Tom Michelsen, who captures the essence of the principles and the process described. This work is for all of you seeking knowledge about the Self in its work of helping others. We offer it to you with Love.

Jacquelyn Small
Rolf Tom Michelsen

P.S. A special thanks to Catherine Lee, Donna Lynn, Nancy and Jimmy at Bear Creek Studios, and Mark Blumenthal for their invaluable input and support.

1. INTRODUCTION

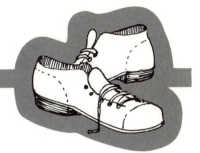

Regardless of your role in life—be it professional therapist, parent, supervisor, or friend—there are ten personal characteristics which correlate with high effectiveness as a therapeutic person in the life of someone else. These ten characteristics correlate with helping (versus actually hindering) another person regardless of your theoretical orientation if you have been trained as a professional therapist. From Freud to existential encounter, these personality variables remain constant. On a scale ranging from 1 to 5, when rating counselors in empirical counselor studies, people who score as high as 3 on these variable scales are "high functioning" therapeutic individuals. People who score 2 or below can actually be harmful agents in any type of interpersonal relationship.

These personal characteristics have been found to correlate with a wide variety of criteria of client improvement, including psychological tests, time out of institutions, clients' self reports, therapist and supervisor ratings, and—even independently—a person will list these characteristics in some form when reporting what type of person he will seek out as a helper. These ten variables hold constant regardless of the diagnostic nature of your client's problem. They have been tested with groups of alcoholics, schizophrenics, delinquents, college counselees, and many other definable groups.

Emerging now from eight years of extensive research in the field of psychotherapy, these counselor variables can be a useful guide for alcoholism counselors as they attempt to look at themselves as helpers in the life of someone else. Those wishing to improve their counseling skills can benefit from a thorough understanding of these traits in action vis-a-vis an alcoholic client. By a thorough understanding, I do not mean merely a "knowing about" these traits, but more a "knowing in your bones", which would include knowledge on the counselor's cognitive, behavioral and emotional levels of being.

From my own experience as a counselor, and my observations of the many beautiful therapists I have encountered in my experiences, I will attempt to dynamically describe these characteristics in a way that can hopefully bring them alive to the reader. For those of you who are already using your naturally therapeutic skills well, you will recognize yourselves in action—give or take a little bit for the unique style each of us possesses. Becoming aware that you have these characteristics, either budding or full-blown, can be an exciting experience. Training programs designed around the experiential development or discovery of these personal traits is an even more exciting prospect, because studies are beginning to indicate that a person can build upon his ability to be a therapeutic individual: we are not creatures "fixed in cement," but are instead dynamic, fluid processes, capable of growth and change at any point.

The Therapeutic Variables. The therapeutic person's characteristics we will explore in detail are empathy, genuineness, respect, self-disclosure, warmth, immediacy, concreteness, confrontation, potency and self-actualization.

Many years ago, a very wise supervisor told me to remember always: "Good counseling is made up of two very, very simple words that just happen to take a lifetime to fully comprehend—*support* and *challenge*." One without the other can be helpful, but will seldom be sufficient to produce growth in a therapeutic relationship. The late Dr. Nathan Ackerman, one of the world's most brilliant family therapists, claimed that counseling is not a skill but an art—that being a good therapist is more like a way of being rather than a set of learned techniques. Anyone can memorize by rote a given set of techniques, but the key to therapeutic relating lies in the mystery of the relationship. Somewhere within the person being the helper and the person being helped something unites and creates a new phenomenon—not a **summation** of parts but an **integration** of a whole. This process is the mystery, delight and pain of self-actualization. And it is a two-way process: the counselor changes and grows along with the client. Sounds rather vague and mystical, doesn't it?

In looking over the therapeutic variables that have emerged from the much less mystical world of empirical research, we can see quickly that these characteristics that correlate with effective counseling do indeed break down into three fairly separate categories: supportive, challenging, and a total way of being. Empathy, genuineness, respect, self-disclosure and warmth can be viewed as basically supportive in their feeling tone, while immediacy, confrontation and concreteness are a way of challenging a person to be more real, truthful and specific in his exploration of himself. Potency and self-actualization (when better understood after careful study) become variables that measure a counselor's overall manner and attitude toward life as he relates to his client and to other significant people in his world.

Support must precede challenge. A warm, supportive, genuine climate must exist before the client will feel enough trust in you to move into the real problem areas of his life, and before he can read your challenging messages as helpful. This is especially true of the alcoholic client, who automatically expects the people in his world to despise him.

In the pages that follow, we will concentrate first on the "supportive" variables, then move on into the later or deeper stages of good counseling by looking at the "challenging" aspects of the relationship, and finally, we can try to capture the flavor of the therapist who is "potent" and "self-actualizing."

The question we are dealing with is this: Can something as artistic, mystical and creative as therapeutic relating be taught as **skill** development? If good counseling is indeed dependent upon such ill-defined phrases as "a total way of being" or "just being naturally therapeutic", what on earth do we attempt to teach?

My conviction is that we have entered again into a paradox (a word which seems to most aptly describe life anyway). Just as an acorn has the innate potential to become an oak tree, we, by just naturally being ourselves, have the inherent ability to be creative and therapeutic. If anything, we have trained **out** of ourselves our naturally therapeutic skills—by becoming (often of necessity) frightened, careful, defensive, closed up, and sometimes even rigid and unbending. Good counselor training may just involve a mere "letting go" again and being naturally what we were intended to be in the first place—before we got so scared.

Note: In the following pages, words that have a technical meaning in the field of psychotherapy are italicized. They are listed in alphabetical order in the Glossary with additional explanation.

Note about the practice exercises: An exercise has been designed at the end of each section to enable you to respond to an alcoholic client mainly by the use of the variable under discussion. It will be helpful if you will make a mental note of your **very first reaction** to this hypothetical client before you begin to experiment with possible ways you might choose to respond. This is the first step in discovering or developing a trait we want to possess or rid ourselves of—becoming aware of what it is we do **now** before we set out to expand or change it.

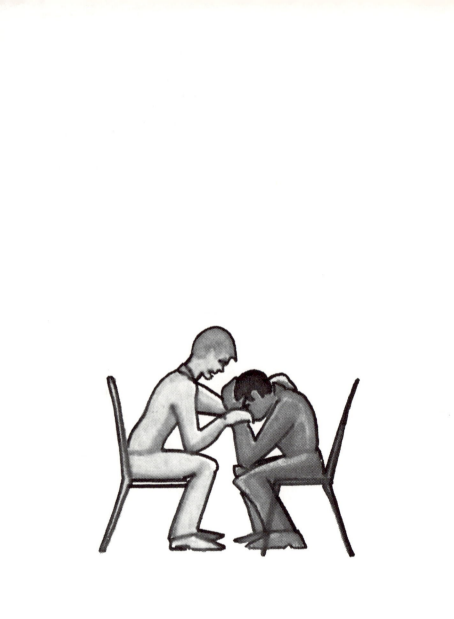

2. EMPATHY

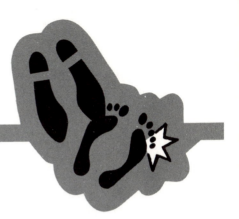

Description. The ability to perceive another's experience and then to communicate that perception back to the individual. As counselor, I listen to you as you speak to me, and though I cannot experience your experience, I begin to have a mind-picture of the essence of what you are describing. I share this with you in "I" language (statements about **me** rather than you).

Empathy-in-action.

Client: (head down, arms crossed, squeezing his chest in a constricted fashion) I just can't .... (sighing) .... can't seem to take it. They all want me to .... oh, I don't see how I can ....

Counselor: I hear you saying your life with your family is strangling you .... some sort of struggle for breath is what I am sensing. I see you looking sad and desperate, with your fists clinched .... and your breath seems constricted as you talk about it. Am I hearing you correctly?

As I talk, I have drawn closer to my client, animated and involved in what I am feeling and attempting to communicate. I even imitate his behavior at times during this interchange, in the way I have perceived it.

Process. This is the process of Empathy-in-action. I have attempted to get "out of my head" (analyzing or interpreting) and just experience in the here and now the essence of my client. I have listened for the "process" instead of hearing only the "content" of his message: I have listened to the whole person within the context of his own unique existence, rather than listening to just his words. I listen to the non-verbal behavior, and the messages I think I read under the surface of his words. As I begin to capture a strong feeling of understanding, I become more active in the session and move in-

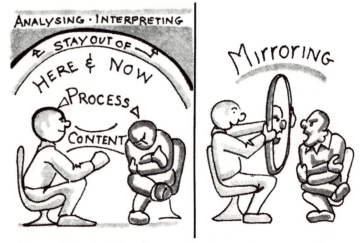

to sharing this with him. I am *reflecting* and *mirroring* for my client—meaning that I feed back to him what I notice. We think we know ourselves so well, but usually, we know our best friend better than we know ourselves. Often, we are not aware of our verbal or non-verbal behavior patterns and messages, until someone points them out to us. Reflecting and mirroring are two techniques that are natural to the involved counselor—and are extremely clarifying maneuvers for the client. In the above example of Empathy-in-action, I am also imparting *non-judgmental feedback*—telling him what I experience in relation to him, using "I" statements—statements about myself rather than about my client: "I hear you saying ...." "I see you looking ....", etc. Non-judgmental feedback is an important concept in counseling, because the client is free to accept or reject what you are perceiving. He does not take your statements as **facts** about him that he must defend against, or accept. Instead, they are statements about **you** in relation to him, which are always truthful statements. I cannot know the facts about your experience, but I can tell you the facts and feelings about how I perceive your experience.

Empathy-in-action is often quite graphic and expresses itself in fantasy images. Notice the counselor's graphic depiction of "strangling" and "constriction." The counselor's mind-pictures match the client's non-verbal behavior, and when fed back to the client in such a dramatic manner, they can serve as a clarifier of unexamined feelings on the part of the client.

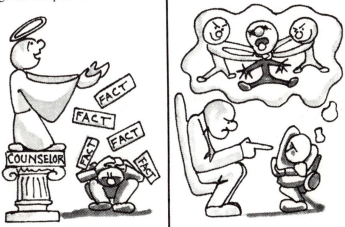

As a counselor, my perceptions may be wrong. I am not ever an expert on another's life. This point cannot be stressed enough. **He** is the only true expert on himself. If I am wrong in my perceptions, my client will tell me in some way by his behavior: He will either say to me directly that I am off, or he will simply not pick up on what I am saying. If I am on target, my client may gain a new understanding of his situation. I have created the possibility for a therapeutic moment by the use of Empathy. I am only one side of the equation, however; I can be wrong, or my client can reject my perceptions even if I am right. He is free to do so. The healing element in operation here is not my correct or incorrect perceptions, but my intense involvement with my client. The communication that is important is taking place on a subterranean, therapeutic level.

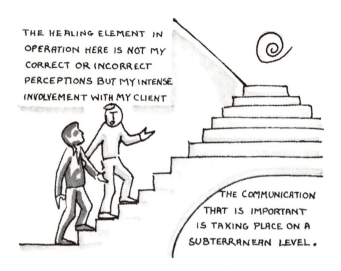

THE HEALING ELEMENT IN OPERATION HERE IS NOT MY CORRECT OR INCORRECT PERCEPTIONS BUT MY INTENSE INVOLVEMENT WITH MY CLIENT

THE COMMUNICATION THAT IS IMPORTANT IS TAKING PLACE ON A SUBTERRANEAN LEVEL.

Opposite of Empathy-in-action. Some examples of the opposite of this variable in operation might be:

1) a counselor who restates to the client the counselor's own perceptions and *projections* as **facts** about the client—which confuses a client and takes him further away from his own reality.

2) a counselor who analyzes a client's situation or dynamics as though he is (or could be) the expert on the client's own inner experience; or

3) a counselor who is not present with the client in the here and now—not free to "be with the client where he is" because he is instead having to use his energy handling his own needs. Perhaps this needs elaboration, because it happens so often.

The inability to really be with a client in the present happens most often when the counselor is clutched about *unfinished business* of his own during the session; or, when the counselor has a great need to be right and uses his energy "laying his theories on" the client and attempting to prove them to him; or, when the counselor spends a great deal of time talking about or listening to the client's past history—content "away off out there somewhere," which can be an avoidance mechanism to keep away from painful here and now material.

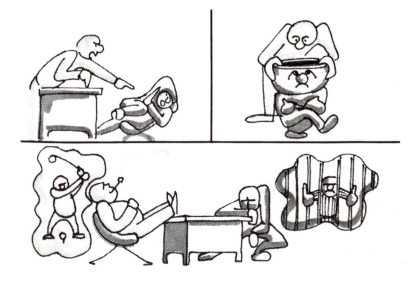

Implications for the alcoholic client. The use of Empathy-in-action enables the alcoholic to feel your presence with him and your sincere interest in trying to discover what his reality is like. As I have mentioned earlier, your perceptions which you share with your alcoholic client may be incorrect; they may be perceptions about **you** that you are projecting onto him, or you just may have heard him wrong. This is not important as long as you state perceptions as perceptions and facts as facts. But you will notice that as you begin to feel free to be with your client in the here and now, you will be amazingly close to his reality as you attempt to share with him your understanding of his world. The therapeutic agent operating with your alcoholic client is your committed **attempt** at understanding your client. His sensing that you care so much—so intently—and are not afraid to get involved with him—is the healing factor. This idea is so simple, yet so very difficult for most counselors to grasp. So many of us tend to become tangled up in trying to be right. Correct interpretations and perceptions can be helpful—sometimes—but more healing than any correct interpretation is your committed attitude of genuine empathy. And having to be right can be extremely unhelpful. Experienced alcoholism counselors report most often that the **one** thing the alcoholic talks of needing the most is to be understood. You may be the first person in his entire drinking years to really try to understand him. The impact of Empathy-in-action on his battered self-esteem will be profound and healing.

A Practice Exercise for you. Practice how you would use Empathy-in-action in the following situation:

Client: After I've had my second or third drink, I begin talking to myself about not drinking any more. Can you imagine that? Talking to myself!! I go back and forth, back and forth. I put the bottle down, walk outside, talk to myself, **cuss** at myself, on and on. (sigh) Then I wind up saying I'll just have one more .... and well, ... there I go .... down into the deep pit again, sometimes not even waking up again for days (puts head down in his hands)

Counselor:

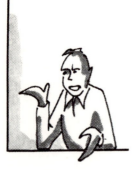

NOTES:

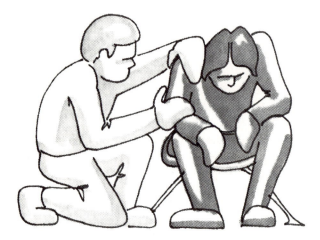

3. GENUINENESS

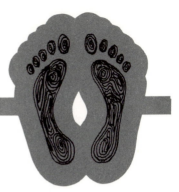

Description. The ability of a counselor to be freely himself—non-phoniness, non-role playing, non-defensiveness. His outer words and behavior match his inner feelings.

Genuineness-in-action.

Client:	(fighting back tears) I'm just not going to think about it anymore .... losing the kid and all .... it's just useless to think about it!
Counselor:	(moves closer to client, touching him on the arm, obviously deeply moved) Johnny, I'm feeling very sad, too, about what happened to your son and seeing your deep, deep hurt.
Client:	(breaks down and weeps)
Counselor:	(quietly shares this moment with client, responding non-verbally like a nurturing parent)

Process. The counselor ignored the defensiveness of the client (the "tough" facade) and moved in as a human being, responding with his real feelings of the moment in a way that kept the client in touch with his real feelings of grief and hurt, rather than taking him away from these and responding to the "pretended" strength. The result was therapeutic: *catharsis* and another small step toward completing an unfinished grief process. Unexpressed grief or anger take up a tremendous amount of psychic and physical energy. If we could see this energy in action, it would literally be a forced holding-in, like two arms crossed and fists clenched, pressing our stomach against our backbone. As long as the energy is being used in this way, it is not free to flow toward the actual solving of problems in daily life, either mentally or physically. Griefwork is a natural process, following a certain pattern from start to finish when we experience a significant loss of any kind. The client must release his anger and his hurt in a natural manner so that he can go on and say goodbye to the lost person or situation and become free again for a life devoid of the loved or needed one. Though grief is natural, it is human to try to avoid it, because **felt** grief is painful. If the people in his environment assist him in running from these natural feelings, *morbid grief* can set in, which manifests itself in several types of unhealthy symptoms.

Opposite of Genuineness-in-action. Many counselors believe they must stay in a professional role when working with a client. Unfortunately, psychoanalytic theory has supported this notion for years by training psychiatrists to remain objective, never touch a patient, keep their own personality out of the way while the patient free associates in a prone position with no eye contact with the doctor. A counselor with this professional mind-set would have said to Johnny, in the above example, something like this: "I understand your feelings, Johnny. Now, what was it you wanted to talk about today?"

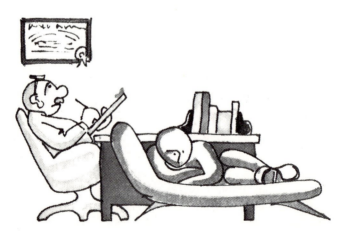

This action would have reinforced Johnny's defenses against feeling the uncomfortable pain of grief, moving him away from his real experience into a distance-keeping, task-oriented discussion. The genuine counselor is not afraid to involve with his client in human feelings that are experienced by all of us. Whether the feelings be sympathy and sadness, anger or joy, the counselor expresses himself with his client in very much the same way he would with a friend outside the counseling relationship. There are some restraints inherent in a counseling relationship that make it different from just a friendship—such as limited contact, lack of social engagement, lack of opportunity for a romance, etc. But these restraints are **real**, not phony. Consequently, counselors never have to fear being real with their clients. If the reality between you is that you cannot stand each other, then the relationship should be terminated anyway. A counselor can never hope to be helpful to someone he really cannot stand to be around. If there is some negative feeling of this type that the counselor or client cannot work through, the relationship is rightfully terminated and an appropriate referral is made. The same holds true for romantic or sexual feelings. If such feelings on either side cannot be worked through after every effort, the relationship should not continue under the strains of a counselor/client situation.

Implications for the alcoholic client. Genuineness is crucial in alcoholism counseling. An alcoholic client will not remain in counseling with a phony, role-playing counselor. Due to his life history, an alcoholic is more sensitive to non-verbal messages and unauthentic behavior than many non-alcoholics are. He expects to be despised and misunderstood. He projects his own bad self feelings onto others, especially persons in authority over him. It is crucial that he learn very early that you are one person who will risk being real with him. If you are angry or hurt by his treatment of you, you must claim these feelings to him openly with "I" statements. He will know how you feel anyway. Remember, he is a master at masking feeling, having learned the hard way all his drinking life. By being yourself, you enable him to make contact with you. Real contact with another individual is the most beautiful gift you can give an alcoholic person.

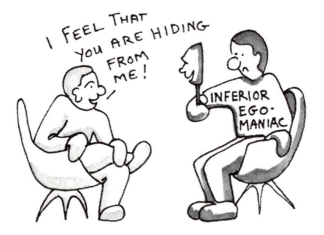

A Practice Exercise for you. Practice how you would respond in a genuine way with the following alcoholic client:

Client: How've you been anyway? Thought I'd stop by. I stood you up for the last couple of times, but you know how it goes .... sometimes it gets ....

Counselor:

N O T E S :

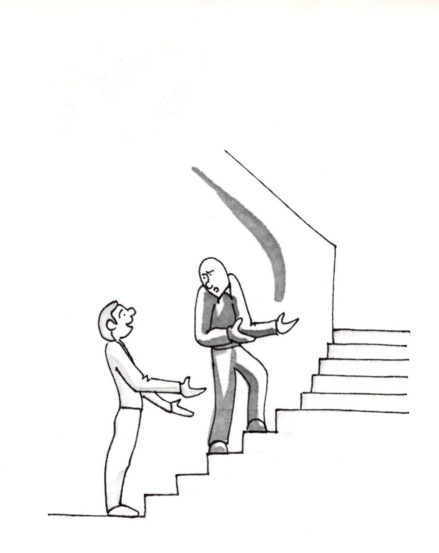

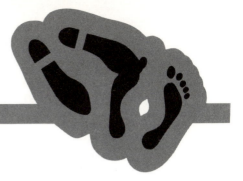

4. RESPECT

Description. The counselor's ability to communicate to the client his sincere belief that every person possesses the inherent strength and capacity to make it in life, and that each person has the right to choose his own alternatives and make his own decisions.

Respect-in-action.

Client: I just want to divorce my wife and get busy forgetting about the whole mess! .... But I can't do it. I really need to stay in there and take care of her .... But I can't seem to do that either. Whew, the whole thing's just got me trapped. What do you think I ought to do .... divorce her?

Counselor: (concerned) Golly, Bill, I can tell you're torn in two on this. Sounds like there's one part of you that needs to stay, but another part of you that wants to get out for good.

Client: Yeh. That's sure it alright.

Counselor: Could you go on and talk for awhile about that part that wants to get out? What does that part of you feel like?

Client: It feels like ....

Counselor: Just a minute, Bill, say instead "I feel like ...." instead of "It." Start your sentences with "I." Go ahead now.

Client: Okay. I FEEL TRAPPED. I want out.

Counselor: Go on, Bill, go on now. Put your **feelings** into what you're saying.

Client:	(getting agitated) **I** feel trapped ! I FEEL TRAPPED!!! I WANT OUT! REALLY OUT! AWAY FROM THE WHOLE GOD-DAMNED MESS!! (puts head down in hands).
Counselor:	(quiet for awhile, allowing the client to absorb his experience) Now, Bill .... (softly) What about that other side of you, the side that needs to stay? Can you talk about that with me a minute?

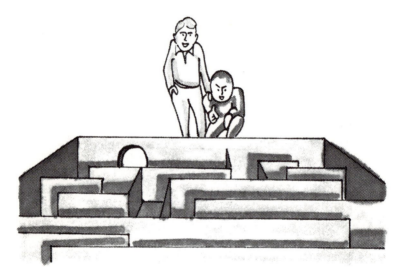

Process. The counselor has not responded to Bill's request to give him the answer to his dilemma, nor to his implied powerlessness in the situation. Instead, he has fed back to the client his observation that the client seems to have two feelings simultaneously. The counselor wants to help the client clarify for himself what each of these sides of him is really feeling. The client thinks he is powerless. Notice, he says "I can't" and "It has got me trapped." Both of these are expressions that say the power is "out there" and I am victim—helpless. By asking the client to talk about each side separately, using "I" statements instead of "it" statements, the counselor is enabling the client to clarify the feelings that reside in each side of himself, and by saying "I" instead of "it" he is staying closer to his real feelings and taking responsibility for them ("**I** feel trapped," rather than "**It** is trapping me"). When a client experiences fully both sides of a split, in the safe counseling environment, he often discovers which side is a "want" and which side is an "I ought to." This can be a clarifying insight that can lead to action. Or he may discover which side contains the most power or which side is really him and which side is merely his **idea** of himself. Once he realizes these feelings more clearly, he is more able to accept both parts of his feelings and make choices for himself that are closer to his own reality. When the energy that has been stored up inside oneself about either side of such a split is released, an amazing kind of integration—or feeling of balance—takes place.

In the above example, the counselor has put the responsibility to make choices back on the client where the power actually resides to make such choices. This is an attitude of respect for the individual, enabling him to discover both his own power and his own responsibility for his decisions in a non-punitive way.

Opposite of Respect-in-action. The most obvious lack of respect-in-action would be if the counselor had attempted to give Bill the answer. "Oh, no, Bill, you don't want to divorce your wife." Or,

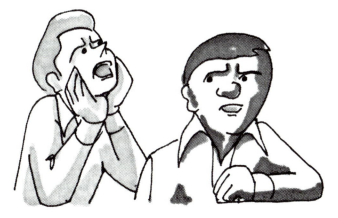

"Well, I wouldn't divorce her if I were you, Bill." Or, if the counselor had ignored the real split feelings going on in Bill and had attempted to preach to him about what he "should" be feeling, the

result would have been unhelpful. In either case, the counselor would have come away "the expert" on Bill's experience, and the client would have missed an opportunity to discover more about his own reality. The client would be further confirmed in his fear that he is powerless and hopeless. ("I can never learn to manage my life like this smart counselor could!")

Implications for the alcoholic client. Respect-in-action helps the alcoholic client take realistic responsibility for himself. A person suffering with alcoholism wavers often between feelings of powerlessness and feelings of omnipotence. Neither extreme is realistic. Respect-in-action does not pamper, nor does it punish. It acknowledges the alcoholic as a person who is learning in his relationship with you what his actual strengths and weaknesses are. You are enabling him to discover these for himself by offering a non-judgmental, clarifying lens through which he can see himself more clearly. Respect-in-action gives the alcoholic hope .... hope that he may actually be a worthwhile individual with the ability to make choices and to govern his own life! Chances are he has gotten out of touch with this possibility.

A Practice Exercise for you. Practice how you would use respect-in-action in the following situation:
Client:

Boy, I've just got to level with my boss about this alcohol problem... But I'm too chicken to do it. I started to 15 times this week, but something stopped me every time — How the Hell can I get up the guts to do it?

Counselor:

NOTES:

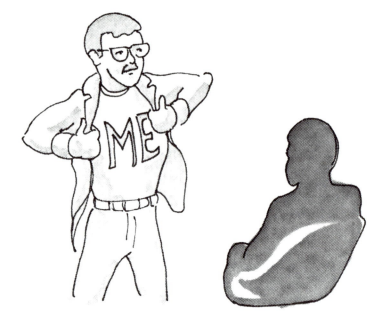

5. SELF-DISCLOSURE

Description: This is the act of sharing and exposing the counselor's own feelings, attitudes and experiences with a client for the sake of the client. Self-disclosure must be meaningful and pertinent both in content and context in order to be therapeutic. It is used with discretion—an accurate sense of timing and appropriateness, with some idea of how the client will make use of the material. It is never used for the counselor's own need to confess or cathart.

Self-disclosure-in-action.

Client: (crying) I just can't let my wife see me like this .... she would think I'm such a stupid weakling!

Counselor: (moving closer to client, with tenderness) I know how you feel, Joe. I have a lot of trouble letting my wife see me when I'm hurting. When I do, I feel weak and stupid, too. I've been told all my life that men are strong, and they don't cry .... haven't you?

Client: (still crying, silently nods)

Counselor: I'm trying to learn to share this scared side of me with Susan. I've been able to do it a few times. And, you know, it's amazing to me, but when I do, she seems to really understand. In fact, we always seem to feel a lot closer to each other after I've been that open with her. I think it somehow must make me more human in her eyes .... or more **with** her, or something.

Client: (looks up, with mild surprise in his voice) You mean **you** really feel like this sometimes, too?

Process. This self-disclosure on your part has helped the client feel acceptable as a human being. He discovers he is not so different from you—that you, too, have problems and make mistakes. Self-disclosure dissolves the "over-under" relationship of the judge and the judged. The client can begin seeing you as another human being, which is reality, rather than as his fantasy of the perfect one who has all the answers for himself. Self-disclosure breeds trust and moves a counseling relationship to deeper levels more quickly. The client will disclose more of the part of himself he is ashamed of or having trouble with. When I don't feel judged by another person, which means I see that person as an equal to me, I feel free to be myself with him, including the parts of me I see as weak or unacceptable.

Opposite of Self-disclosure-in-action. The counselor who can never share anything from his own life with a client is one who has a need to maintain the role of expert, judge or superior person. He will keep his relationship with his client at a safe distance, creating a climate of caution and superficiality, which is non-therapeutic.

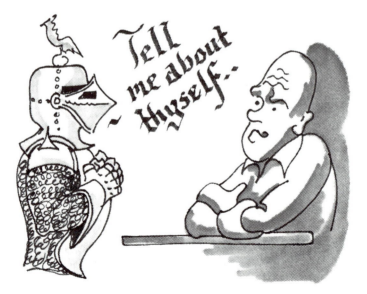

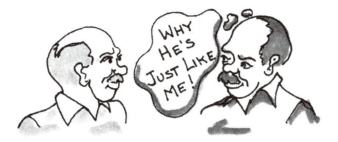

Implications for the alcoholic client. Self-disclosure on the part of the counselor enhances the alcoholic's ability to test having an intimate relationship with someone, a form of *corrective emotional experience:* He is terribly deficient in the area of intimate relationships—a deficiency which is both a cause and an effect of his drinking.

Sometimes it is easier to comprehend the alcoholic's felt reality if you can think of his drinking years as having been a time period when his socialization process came to a grinding halt. While living through his years of alcoholic drinking, he has literally "buried himself in a bottle." His entire life has become "alcohol centered;" the result has been a paucity in every other area of his life. He is practicing and learning only two skills well: how to protect and maintain his supply, and how to rationalize his behavior to others in order to maintain the remnants of his self respect. His job, his marriage, his friendships, his talents and dreams—all have been tainted or have become non-existent during his drinking years. If the alcoholic drinking has lasted for ten years, he may have ten years' socialization skills to catch up on once a fairly steady sobriety has been achieved. A non-drinking alcoholic and a non-alcoholic may walk into a room of strangers together and both may appear at ease—but chances are the non-alcoholic knows what to do in this social situation, while the alcoholic may be feeling anxiety-ridden and completely at sea.

I am generalizing at this point about "alcoholics" and "non-alcoholics," which makes me somewhat uncomfortable, because in most instances this is a false distinction; however, I am contending that alcoholic behavior does produce some **direct** consequences which must not be overlooked in the counseling relationship. Your ability to disclose yourself in a deeply personal manner will enable your client to practice in a safe relationship some interpersonal sharing that may be extremely useful to him in his other relationships as he learns to relate without the comforting support of alcohol.

A Practice Exercise for you. The client situation described below affords a counselor the opportunity to disclose himself to this client in a helpful manner. Practice how you would respond.

Client: I sure don't look forward to weekends at my house .... oh, dear, that's a terrible thing to say. I didn't mean that I don't love my family. I really do love my kids very much. I know they are little, and bless their little hearts, **they** can't help it if they need me all the time. I just mean .... well, never mind.

Counselor:

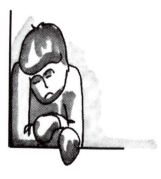

N O T E S :

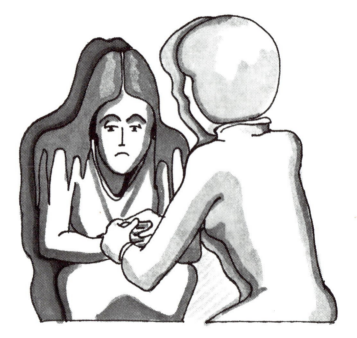

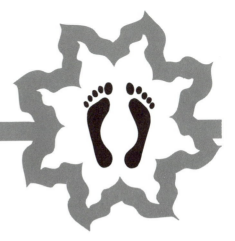

6. WARMTH

Description. Warmth is a characteristic evident mainly from the non-verbal communication of the counselor toward the client. Behaviors, such as smiles, touching and other natural responses to the humanness of the client are evidence of Warmth-in-action. Even tears shed appropriately with a client who is suffering a loss are considered therapeutic.

Warmth-in-action.

Client: (crying and rocking back and forth, holding her hands tensely in her lap) Ever since John died, I've felt so lost and .... and untouched. Sometimes it's just unbearable. I just die to be touched sometimes.

Counselor: (Leans forward and takes client's hands, and as she does so, the client falls into counselor's arms. Counselor holds client for awhile, in silence, gently rocking client to and fro, stroking her hair.)

Process: The above described scene would have received a highly negative response from traditionally-trained counselors or supervisors, having been viewed as dangerous and a violation of the therapeutic process. Based mainly on Freudian psychology, we have been trained to believe the therapist should remain objective and unemotional within the confines of the counselor/client relationship. Research, however, shows otherwise: Clients need touching. They need to feel the counselor's humanness. We are asking our clients to open up with us, and to share their deepest feelings, hopes and fears. Consequently, we must model this ability to be open and responsive—thus allowing the client to feel what she feels without any awkwardness.

In the above example, the client was attempting to nurture herself by rocking to and fro. Observing this behavior, the counselor chooses to become the nurturer herself and takes over the rocking as a mother might. The counselor remains silent to give the client space to **feel** without having to deal with comments from the counselor. It is therapeutic for the client to stay with her feelings of loneliness and need, and to go on through the feelings honestly. The fact that the counselor responded to the desire for nurturing teaches the client that life outside will respond to her when she asks for something. This is a subtle, non-verbal message of hope.

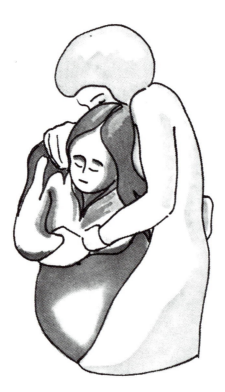

Opposite of Warmth-in-action. A counselor low in Warmth operates from an injunction against showing feelings too openly. This injunction may have come from an original family life in which there was little touching. In such families, children grow up learning to hold back their touching responses with others. Or the training of the counselor may have mandated a "professional attitude" of emotional non-involvement

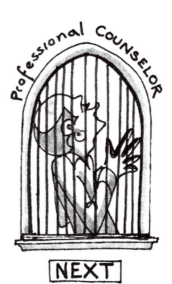

with clients. In either case, the counselor would be uncomfortable with responding to the client, as the counselor in our example. Instead, this counselor would either intellectualize, discount the client's pain or freeze.

Intellectualizing:

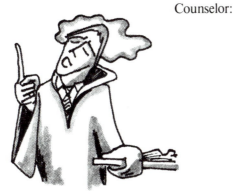

Counselor: It's natural that you would miss John a great deal, Sarah. You have just begun the grief process. Can you tell me, how long have you been feeling this terrible loneliness?

This response would put the client "in her head" to analyze her behavior and check out her recent history of dealing with the loss of her husband. It could produce some insight, but it will not aid her in moving through the grief process in a natural and healing way. Catharsis and learning to reach out for nurturing are much more therapeutic for this client.

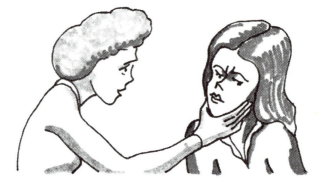

Discounting:

Counselor: Now, Sarah, you act as though you think no other man in the world will ever pay attention to you! Why, you are a beautiful lady. You will have another meaningful relationship soon, I'm sure.

This type of response is premature and irrelevant at this stage of the grief process. This client is nowhere near ready to begin thinking of other relationships, and reassuring her of her desirability is extremely inappropriate at this time. Still stuck in the past, she is not ready to look ahead ... and rightfully so, for there is still griefwork to be done.

Freezing: When a counselor freezes, it is apparent she has been confronted with a human situation with which she is not prepared emotionally to deal. Her behavior will appear awkward and irrelevant—not coming from the same emotional level as the client. Any type of freezing behavior shuts a client down for the moment, causing her to pull back, change the subject or become silent.

Clients often mirror for us what we are allowing them to feel. They will most often follow your lead.

A Note to counselors who feel they are not naturally warm. If your demeanor is reserved and display of feelings and touching are uncomfortable for you, please do not feel you must force yourself to develop the natural ability to express Warmth. It is far better to be yourself, and continue developing Genuineness with your clients. If you are genuine and learn to self-disclose a little, you will find you can share with your client at an appropriate time that you would like to display more affection with them but it is not natural to you. This type of rapport will build a type of Warmth that is a very special form of Genuineness.

A Special Note about seduction. Natural human Warmth is not seductive, nor is it interpreted as a mixed message by your client. Holding, touching and intimate sharing are human qualities that surface during times of suffering and need. The "vibration" is different from the counselor who is being sexual or seductive. Warmth can easily be expressed between male and female counselor/client. It will, if anything, serve as a safety against seductiveness. You may need to experience this to believe me.

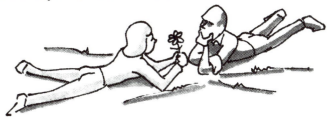

Implications for the alcoholic client. A major hurdle toward a stable sobriety is this client's ability to deal with her feelings appropriately. Fear of feelings is a lot of what alcoholism is all about. One drinks to hide feelings, or to handle negative feelings such as anxiety, nervousness, uncertainty or fear. When an alcoholic client begins to risk showing real feelings with you, the more authentically you can respond, the better therapist you are.

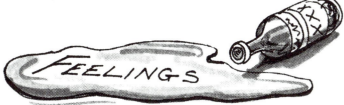

A Practice Exercise for you. This client is a male, very rigid and afraid of contacting others. He has been raised in a non-touching "chauvinistic" family that views emotional sharing as a form of weakness. He is losing his wife through divorce, and the feelings of sadness are just underneath the surface.

Client: (Looking scared and childlike) I've never known whether or not it was okay to ask someone to hold me .... I mean, sometimes I just would like to be held like a little baby or something. But, it's not like me, I mean, I wouldn't know how, or what to do ....

Counselor:

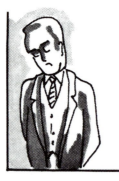

NOTES:

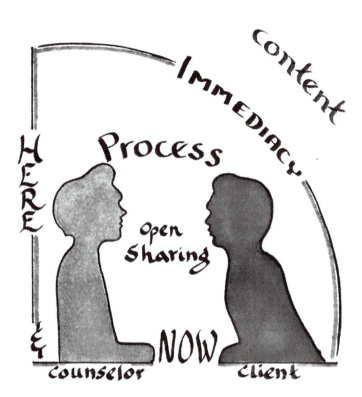

content

Immediacy

HERE

Process

Open Sharing

&

NOW

counselor

client

7. IMMEDIACY

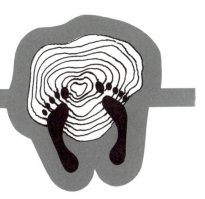

Description. This variable is dealing with the feelings between the counselor and the client in the here and now—an open sharing of what is going on between you and your client right now. This therapeutic method takes the emphasis off the content of the client's problems "out there" and places it on the process going on in the room between the two of you.

Immediacy-in-action

A. Immediacy when the feelings of the moment are negative:

Counselor: I'm beginning to feel uncomfortable right now, Jerry, because I'm sensing that you are very angry with me and not wanting to talk with me about it. Are you mad at me?

Client: Well, not exactly .... but .... well, I **do** feel like you're not listening to me today. It seems like your mind is on something else .... or you're not interested in me .... or something.

Counselor: (pauses to reality-check this feedback with himself) You know, you're absolutely right, Jerry. I can see why you're mad. I really **am** distracted. In fact .... yeah, in **fact**, I'm annoyed with you for not showing up yesterday, and I'm really not wanting to listen to you today .... like, it's my way of getting back at you. Yeah .... I'm aware of it now. I'm mad as heck at **you**!! I think we better deal with this first.

Process. Counselors are not totally self-actualized people, either. Often, a counselor is not himself "all together" or "in touch with his feelings." In this example, the counselor has projected his own anger onto the client, and until he asks for the client's feedback, he has not himself become aware of this. But he **was** aware that the session was not getting anywhere. By the use of Immediacy, they will go ahead

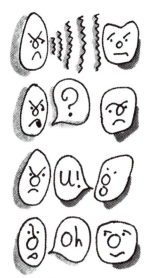

and confront the feelings that were dwelling underneath the surface, cluttering up their ability to be real with each other. By getting all this out in the open, the feelings will dissolve, and they will be free to explore together the client's work at hand. The counselor has modeled for the client how to reality-test and attempt bringing communication to a genuine level of involvement. They are bringing their honest feelings to the level of awareness so they can be dealt with.

B. Immediacy when the feelings of the moment are positive:

Client: I've brought you a little present today .... it's not much .... but it's something I wanted to give to you.

Counselor: (deeply moved) Thank you, Nancy. I am very touched by this. I'm feeling very strongly right now that you do care a lot about me. Is that what you're feeling?

Client: (blushes and smiles, self-consciously) Uh huh ....

Counselor: (grins broadly) Well, I do feel **good** hearing that!! I care very deeply for you, too, Nancy. In fact, I think you are a neat gal, you know it?!! I really **like** you!!

Client:	(embarrassed, but obviously very pleased) Well, golly .... You're saying that .... Well, you're saying that .... You **really mean** that? I don't know when I've .... (suddenly begins to weep)
Counselor:	(allows client to assimilate this very intimate moment by quietly sitting with her as she goes on and feels moved. When Nancy begins to come out of the feeling ....) You seemed so moved by this, Nancy. I guess you're pretty starved out for good friends, huh?
Client:	Yeah, I think I am. I don't know **when** I've felt close to anyone .... (weeps again) .... and I really **want** to. (puts head down)
Counselor:	(very softly) Well, tell me something. What could you do about that? Does anything occur to you?
Client:	You mean .... in my day-to-day life?
Counselor:	Yes, that's what I mean. What could you do about this feeling of being so starved out?

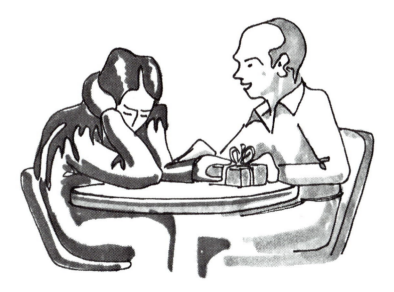

Process. The counselor, by dealing with the immediate process (their sincere caring for each other), has kept the client close to her reality. By sharing honestly with the client, he enabled her to be herself in a direct manner. (The giving of the gift was an **indirect,** less satisfactory means of saying that she cared and wanted the counselor's approval.) The encounter with reality on the feeling level moved them to a very productive interchange that invited the client to experience genuine caring in a safe environment, plus inviting her to look honestly at a crucial part of her life: What can she do to develop closer relationships with people—or how she is blocking herself from fulfilling this vital need?

In both the above instances of Immediacy-in-action, an honest exchange of genuine intimacy served as a laboratory experience for them to learn how to give and receive honest anger or affection in a manner that leads to satisfaction. This is significant learning that can lead to growth.

Opposite of Immediacy-in-action. Immediacy is one of the most threatening techniques of therapeutic involvement for the counselor and the client. Practice and learning to tolerate a certain amount of anxiety are necessary in order to build this characteristic. In the first example, it would have been much safer for the counselor to ignore the hostility he was feeling in his client and in himself as they were attempting to get into the session. The counselor would have kept a safe distance from his client, and would have allowed him to continue discussing whatever was on the surface. Nothing very productive would have happened, but the

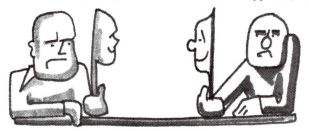

counselor **could** have maintained safety in his role of "being on top of it," and the client would not have had to face his counselor's possible rejection by claiming his feeling that the counselor was not listening to him. A defensive, unaware counselor would have denied that he was angry with his client, and consequently, the client would have become even more angry with him for having suggested that the counselor may not have been listening to him.

In the second example, if the counselor had merely said thank you for the gift and moved the session on into a discussion about something other than the process in the here and now, the client would not have experienced what it is like to share intimately in a direct way with another human being—nor would she have encountered so vividly her real feelings of paucity in relationships. Her indirect, apparently unsatisfactory pattern of showing affection (gift giving) would have been reinforced and no new learning would have occurred.

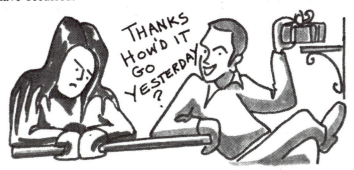

Implications for the alcoholic client. Most alcoholics live in a world of disassociation from their own feelings. By the overuse of *unconscious denial* and *projection* as protective devices, they have usually recreated their reality in a way that they can live more comfortably. But, unfortunately, this very maneuver which is used to produce comfort usually produces more discomfort, as their reconstructed reality is constantly out of tune with what is really going on in their lives. The use of Immediacy can help the alcoholic client relearn (or learn) how to look at his own feelings and the feelings of his counselor in the safety of the counseling relationship.

The rewards of being accepted for one's real self are so great, and the relief of expressing what is actually going on inside is so gratifying, that the alcoholic client will benefit from this practice immensely as time goes by and he begins to trust his experience more—and his fantasies less.

A Practice Exercise for you. In the following example, there is something going on under the surface that is getting in the way of a productive counseling session. See how you would respond with Immediacy-in-action.

Client: (laughing self-consciously) Well, I had this dream last night that you and I were in this boat. (pauses) Yeah, it was you alright .... and we were in the water, and the waves were getting higher and higher, oh this is so silly .... but .... and I kept hanging on to you, and you got bigger and bigger .... in fact you actually became a **balloon** .... sort of a **life** raft or something .... (pauses, looking helplessly and self-consciously at the counselor).

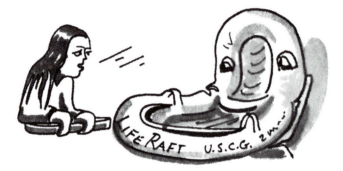

Counselor:

N O T E S :

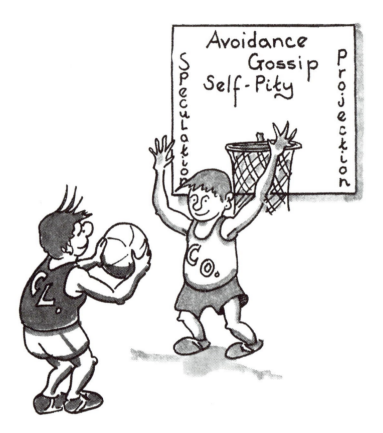

8. CONCRETENESS

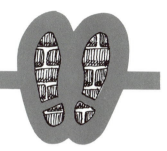

Description: The act of keeping the client's and the counselor's own communications specific—getting to the whats, whens, wheres and hows of relevant concerns. The concrete counselor does not go off on tangents or get into generalizations or abstract discussions with his client. He keeps his client talking about **himself,** and into **his own feelings,** rather than speculating or gossiping about other persons in his life. The counselor who can be concrete has the ability to detect his client's own unique ways of avoiding his reality and the ability to confront these avoidance behaviors by artfully drawing the client back to relevant issues and feelings of the moment.

Concreteness-in-action (when client is generalizing)

Client: Oh well, about the fight with my husband .... well, you know, all husbands and wives seem to have a problem about ....

Counselor: Martha, I'm not interested right now in all husbands and wives. I'm very much interested in what you started to say while ago .... something about you are feeling mad at yourself because of some kind of fight that happened with Mark. Can you go on with that?

Concreteness-in-action (when the client is gossiping)

Client: Marge is always telling me what to do. She feels like she's got to be in the driver's seat all the blasted time! Just like last night. She felt hurt and mad at me because she seems to want some kind of expression of **something** from me ....

Counselor:	George, I'm getting lost in Marge and trying to psyche her out. Where are **you** in all this? What are **you** feeling while Marge is trying to control you? You look very angry right now as you're telling me about last night. What are you feeling?
Client:	Angry?
Counselor:	Yes. You were really scowling as you were talking about Marge just now. You were also clenching your fist.
Client:	(pauses, somewhat confused, but begins clenching fist again)
Counselor:	George, what is this? (mirrors clenched fist gesture)
Client:	(Begins hitting the palm of his hand with his clenched fist) I **hate** it!!! I can't **stand** her always telling me what to do!!! I want to tell her to .... to GO TO HELL!! Yeah, GO TO HELL, MARGE!! GET OFF MY BACK!! I'M AS GOOD AS YOU **ANY** DAY. **ANY** DAY, YOU HEAR?? (As client's anger begins subsiding, he puts his head in his hands and begins breathing deeply.)
Counselor:	What are you feeling now, George?
Client:	Better. (smiles) Yes. Much, **much** better.

Process: In the first instance, when the client is generalizing, Martha is wanting to avoid some unpleasant feelings she is having about a situation which exists between her husband and herself. She is escaping into generalities, which are much easier and safer to deal with than the more scary issue at hand—her bad-self feelings in relation to her husband. The counselor pulls her back to her experience in the moment by being concrete, and the intervention creates an opportunity for a productive session.

In the second example, the client is using gossip about his wife's feelings and inferences about her dynamics to avoid getting in touch with a feeling he imagines to be unacceptable: absolute fury at a "perfect wife and mother." The counselor again manages to draw the client into the much more relevant issue of his own feelings. The client cannot change Marge anyway; he doesn't have the power.

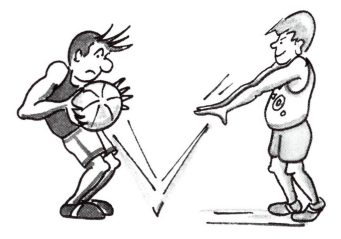

But he **can** have power over what **he** chooses to do in relation to Marge—once he becomes clear on what he wants or needs to do. This particular counseling session was especially fruitful for the client for three reasons: First, it helped to clarify for the client what his real feelings were about Marge's domineering style. Second, by going on into his feelings of fury (via the clenched fist), a lot of stored-up psychic energy became freed to use in more productive ways. And third, George was given permission by his counselor to go ahead and feel fury at his wife and he discovered that his feelings were acceptable after all, and even perhaps natural.

Sometimes a client will continue to avoid an important issue even when the counselor makes efforts at concreteness. If the client is not truly ready to deal with a certain painful area, this need for avoidance must be respected; the need for avoidance may be just as relevant at that particular time as the issue the counselor knows lurks beneath the avoidance behavior. It is always important in counseling that the counselor "be where the client is" in his development and not attempt to jump too far ahead of him. But it is also important to constantly present the client with his here and now reality. In this instance, the reality is that the client is avoiding (maybe for very good reason) and the counselor is getting nowhere by his efforts at concreteness. This observation in the here and now can also be therapeutic: The counselor can claim to the client that he feels *stuck*. (This is the beauty of working in the here and now: everything the counselor observes can be used in therapy.) When a counselor claims very honestly that he is stuck, this puts the responsibility on the client to move the session to some other area of the client's choosing, which often is the client's examination of his own avoidance behavior. In any event, if the process the counselor was trying to reach by concreteness is important in the life of this client, it will recur with frequency, and the client will encounter it when his own inner timing is right.

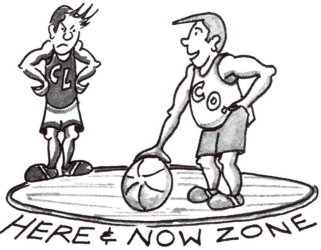

HERE & NOW ZONE

Opposite of Concreteness-in-action. In the first example given, the counselor would have listened to Martha's statement about husbands and wives in general and would have contributed to it by additional generalities of his own: "Yes, it does seem to me that marriages are made up of ..." No one ever grows much by hearing about "people in general." When I am suffering in my relationship with my husband, all other wives and husbands in the world are totally irrelevant to my problem with my husband. At that moment in time, I am unique. I hurt. I'm feeling bad about myself, and I need help with my very own special problem. I may seek to avoid my hurt, and that is my choice—but my counselor is doing me no service to allow me to avoid without my knowledge that I am avoiding. If I did not avoid solving my own problems, I would never need counseling in the first place.

Counselors who have trouble being concrete usually discover that the client controls the session, going on and on about first one thing and then another. This situation can make a counselor feel impotent and exasperated, usually resulting in a desire to avoid this particular client! Counselors often blame the client for this, unknowingly. A more careful look at your ability to be concrete might be illuminating in instances where you feel you are failing with a client.

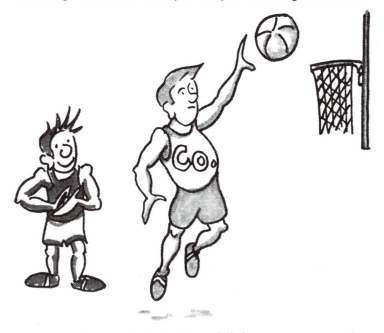

Implications for the alcoholic client. It is important to remember that the alcoholic client usually assumes that no one is interested in him anyway—or that no one really sees him as a person of value. He will generalize and speak "around problems" many times to test out your interest, or just to make conversation. An astute counselor will watch for clues in the alcoholic's conversation that point to problem areas he would really like to discuss with you.

Many alcoholism counselors have noted the alcoholic client's amazing ability to intellectualize (another form of generalizing). It is almost as though this client in particular has a really special need to keep his mind working overtime processing ideas and information. Some recovering alcoholics have told me they are convinced that in their own individual case, this is a way they keep themselves from living in the present. "It is easier for me to trust an **idea** about the world than it is to really experience it," one concerned client said.

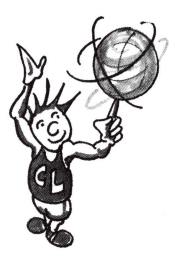

Concreteness in your counseling sessions can be very useful both to help the alcoholic get to his very specific problems and to help **you** communicate your specific interest in him.

A Practice Exercise for you. Practice utilizing the skill of concreteness in the following situation:

Client: Hi, Mary. Golly, I had a hard time getting here today. I went to a party last night, and .... oh, did I tell you my sister is here? We are really having a reunion! Wow! What a reunion! And Joey didn't come by all week, and oh, yes, I wanted to tell you what Dr. Smith said on Tuesday. Golly, this dress of mine is too tight. Whew. Well, anyway, at the party last night I met an old friend. I've told you about all I did when I was in boarding school, didn't I? Well, this friend is from 'way back in those days. Yeah, at that boarding school, we used to sleep in the ....

Counselor:

NOTES:

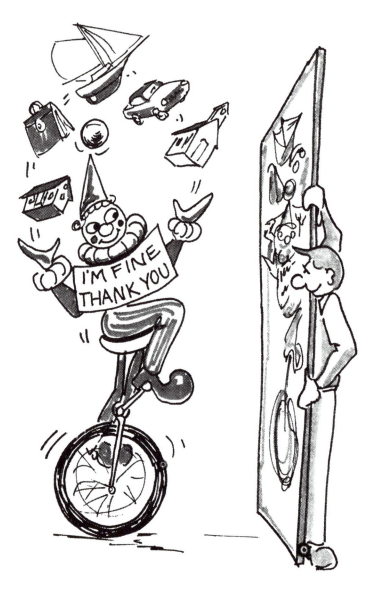

9. CONFRONTATION

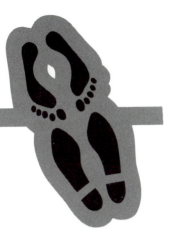

Description. The act of bringing the client face to face with his reality as you perceive him as a whole person. Confrontation occurs when there is an observed discrepancy between:

a) what a client is saying and your perception of what he is experiencing;

b) what he is saying and what you heard him say at an earlier time; or

c) what he is saying now and his actions in his everyday life.

Deciding whether or not to confront a client is always a decision within the counselor's control and is used when he believes it is appropriate. Confrontation can precipitate a crisis point in the client's life, but usually some kind of breakthrough occurs for the client as a result of your therapeutic confrontation. Also, a deeper level of trust grows between you as a result of your having risked this kind of honesty with him. As confronting is difficult for most people, and can be harmful if used inappropriately, more time will be spent in detailing this type of therapeutic encounter. This is the most crucial variable in alcoholism counseling because of the client's extreme use of unconscious denial, rationalization and projection .... or, in the language of Alcoholics Anonymous, "stinking thinking."

Confrontation-in-action. If we very carefully analyse the art of therapeutic confrontation in interaction, we discover there are five types:*

a) **Experiential Confrontation.**

This is an encounter in the here and now, usually occurring when the counselor observes a discrepancy between what the client is saying and what he is apparently experiencing as he says it:

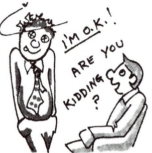

Client: (slightly intoxicated, whiskey on breath) I'm just feeling **awfully** good today!! I'm not even **worried** anymore about controlling **my** drinking! In fact .... I'm ....

Counselor: Ohhh wait a minute, Sue. I'm feeling very uncomfortable with you right now. I'm thinking you had to drink today to boost yourself up just to see ME!!

Client: Oh, now, wait a minute ....

Counselor: No, Sue. Right now you remind me of a little girl scared half to death, feeling miserable, and worried to **death** about your drinking. I don't believe you are feeling good at all. Come on now, Sue. What's going on here with us—here, right now?

b) **Strength Confrontation.**

This type of encounter occurs when the client is "pretending weakness" in an area where the counselor knows or suspects the client has strength:

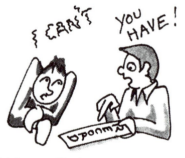

Client: I just don't know how to go about getting another job. (droops in chair) I guess I'm just ....

Counselor: Now Joe, I won't buy that. Just last week you outlined for me very clearly four or five ways you have successfully changed jobs in the past .... and always toward a promotion! Now, come on, Joe. What is this (mirrors his slumped, "pitiful" posture and expression)? What are you doing with this .... here with me now?

c) **Weakness Confrontation.**
When counselor observes a
client "playing tough" to avoid
an obvious difficulty he's having, this type of confrontation
is useful:

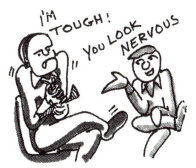

Client: Well let me tell
             you .... She just
             can't get to **me**
anymore with all that cryin' and yellin'. When she
starts up I just tell her to knock it off right then and
there!!

Counselor: (gently) Michael, I'm sorry, but I don't believe you.
             You look "gotten to" even now as you talk about it.
             Your eyes are sad; you're fidgeting in your chair ....
             (leans forward) I believe this problem with Carol is
             still upsetting you very much.

d) **Action Confrontation.** This type of confrontation boosts the
client toward an agreed-upon goal or contract:

Client: Hi, Mr. Johnson.
             Sure glad to get
             out of that ....

Counselor: James, I'm not going to
             keep my appointment
             with you today, and I
             believe you
             already know why.

Client: Well, I ....

Counselor: You look doubtful. Well, Jane Smith from AA called
             me this morning wanting to know if I'd seen you,
             because she hasn't. You and I have a very clear agree-
             ment that I see you if you go to AA. I'm feeling very
             disappointed and annoyed, James, because I've felt
             we're really getting somewhere together. And I'm
             really liking working with you.

Client: Yeah, me too. Aw, come on. Give me another
             chance.

Counselor: Nope. Won't do either of us any good. (rising) I'll see you next week, **if** you get to AA on Thursday. That's your part. I'll keep your appointment time open. It's up to you (terminates session).

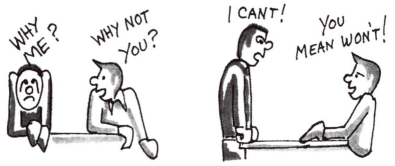

e) **Factual Confrontation.** This method of confronting occurs when the counselor imparts facts to correct the client's imaginings or some misinformation he is operating from.

1. **Example of correcting imaginings.**

Client: You know, when I walk into that classroom everybody in the whole room looks up at me with disgust.

Counselor: Everybody in the room?

Client: Yeah, every one of 'em.

Counselor: That's hard for me to believe, Pete. I've never known of a group of people anywhere who could all be having the same feeling at the same time .... especially about me! I've never known of that many people even being that **interested** in me all at one time .... aren't these people almost total strangers to you?

Client: Yeah .... but it sure seems that way to me.

Counselor: Pete, what could be going on in **you** that makes you feel so bad when you walk in there?

2. **Example of correcting misinformation.**

Client: I can't tell my husband I'm an alcoholic! And I also can't stop drinking completely right now, either. You see ....

Counselor: Just a minute, Joan. You mean you **won't**. There are only three or four things you **can't** do: you can't go without food and you can't go without water;

70

	things like that .... there are so few things you really **can't** change. Now, start over and say "I **won't** tell my husband" and "I won't stop drinking." Tell me you **choose** not to. I want to see **you** take the responsibility for both those decisions. **You're** in control here—not some **thing** "out there" stopping you. Now, (gently) go on ....
Client:	Okay, damnit!!! I **WON'T** tell my husband, and I **WON'T** stop drinking right now! I WON'T, I WON'T! (breaks into tears)
Counselor:	(silent while she assimilates this experience) (tenderly) How are you feeling now, Joan?
Client:	Well, I feel STUPID!! It's like I do these things to myself .... (sobs) over and over again.
Counselor:	Joan! Did you feel the power in you when you were shouting "I WON'T!!"? There was a lot of strength in that .... coming from **you**. What do you want to do with all that power? What are you willing to do?

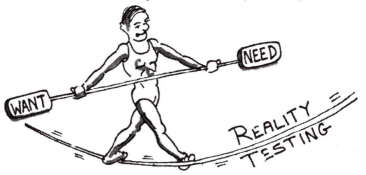

Process. By all the above confrontation examples, the counselor has enabled the client to experience the ways he keeps himself from his own reality and from meeting his own vital needs. *Reality-testing* and learning to take responsibility for his behavior are two vital steps your client must take in order to lead a functional life.

---

*The five types of confrontation listed are an expansion of a suggested classification system devised by group leaders as discussed in *The 1973 Annual Handbook for Group Facilitators,* Pfeiffer and Jones (eds.), University Associates Publishers, Inc., La Jolla, Calif.

The counselor must always check out his own inner feelings as he responds to a client. When he becomes aware that his inner feeling is disbelief or doubt about what the client is expressing, he has the option to confront the client with his perception of what is going on. If a relationship of trust has not been established with a client, the counselor may choose not to confront every discrepancy, or to go easy. His manner and attitude are crucial. If he is non-caring or uninvolved with the client, confrontation can be useless or harmful. Honest, helpful confrontation comes out of a deep trusting relationship—but it **creates** deep and trusting relationships, too. As with all paradoxes, the counselor's own unique use of self within the context with a unique individual must guide him in his choices of confrontation. There are no general rules to guide you, but there are some conditions to look for that tend to make confrontation helpful rather than harmful:

Counselor Conditions:
1. Am I sensitive to the amount of trust and kind of feeling tone that exists between my client and me?
2. Am I willing to become more involved with him as a person?
3. Am I confronting his concrete behavior, something he can really do something about?
4. Am I making my confrontation positive and constructive, rather than negative and punitive?
5. Am I being direct and easily understood?
6. Am I representing facts as facts, feelings as feelings, and inferences as inferences?
7. Have I laid down my cards first? In other words, does he know what is motivating me to confront him?

Client Conditions:
1. Will he accept my confrontation as an invitation to explore himself?
2. Is he open to knowing how he is seen or experienced by others?
3. Can he tolerate some discomfort and mental pain which may result from my confrontation?
4. Does he believe that I care about him?

to Confront or not to Confront that is the ?

If the answer to most of the questions is "yes," favorable conditions exist for helpful confrontation.

Most often we know when a situation **needs** confronting; it is our choice of whether or not to confront **when we see the need** that merits scrutiny. Some choices not to confront are valid; e.g., when we know trust has not developed sufficiently, or when we know too many of the above counselor/client conditions are lacking. Sometimes a client is too emotionally distraught in a certain area to get into a particular set of feelings—timing is very important. But, sometimes we hold back from confronting to protect **ourselves** from something. If we become aware that we are doing this, we must explore ourselves to see what it is we fear. Some of the most common fears about confrontation are the following:

1. Fear of rejection. (I need my client's approval.)
2. Fear of being wrong. (Maybe I'll confront and then I can't prove to my client that I'm right.)
3. Fear of unpleasantness—anxiety, tears, anger. (I just don't know how to act in the face of these emotions.)
4. Fear of intimacy. (Boy, this will bring us face to face with all the barriers down!)

If these kinds of fears are stopping us from confronting a client's messed up picture of reality and belief systems, they are invalid in the therapeutic relationship and must be worked through. A counselor cannot be effective if he is not able to confront. It is important not to confuse being **able** to confront with being **comfortable** with confrontation. Anyone who becomes too comfortable with confrontation would have to be a little too unfeeling to be very therapeutic.

Opposite of Helpful Confrontation. Harmful confrontation results when a counselor has ulterior motives, or a "hidden agenda," of which he himself may not even be aware. Another way of saying this is the counselor may have problems of his own that he works out at his client's expense. Some examples are:

1. A counselor who harbors pent-up hostilities might play what Eric Berne referred to as the "NIGYSOB" game with his client: "Now I've Got You, You Son-of-a-Bitch." Quite frankly, some recovered alcoholic counselors who have not yet forgiven themselves for their drinking history can play this game unwittingly. The confronter carefully watches the confrontee until he catches him in a mistake. He is then justified in venting his anger with some kind of put-down, which he rationalizes by saying "I'm only trying to help you." But let me quickly point out—recovered alcoholic counselors do not hold a monopoly on this well-known game!

2. A counselor who has a need to show off his perception and knowledge can confront in harmful ways that usually sound very clinical and aloof. He will pin on the client diagnostic labels, interpretations and inferences that are of little use to the client, and can be harmful if the client happens to respect the counselor a great deal and "buys" these as facts about himself. Sometimes degreed professionals who are still uncertain about their own professional identity fall into this trap.

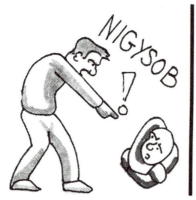
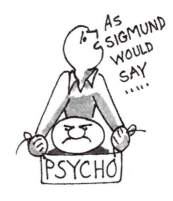

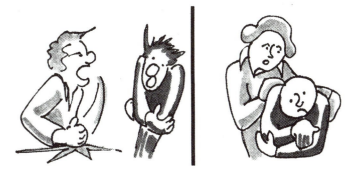

3. Sometimes a counselor will confront just to stir things up a bit—out of a sense of boredom or impotence. The counselor needs to be clear about his motives for confronting.
4. Constantly avoiding obviously needed confrontations can be a harmful type of confrontation in itself! If I treat you constantly with "kid gloves" regardless of your behavior, what message am I really giving you? That I think you are too weak or pitiful to handle the truth about yourself, right? Hardly a therapeutic inference!!

Implications for the alcoholic client. Honest, caring and direct confrontation is the backbone of good counseling for the alcoholic client. Elaborating on the harmful aspects of confrontation may have caused you to feel confrontation should be avoided. Nothing could be further from my intention! Interpersonal confrontation is one of the most potent and therapeutic tools a counselor can work with effectively for someone suffering from alcoholism. Unfortunately, the word confrontation has become a negatively loaded term, carrying harmful connotations—when actually, **helpful** confrontation brings the client into more direct contact with his own experiencing and creates a situation where growth can occur. Nothing could benefit a person on the "merry-go-round of denial" more. But because confrontation **is** such a potent, growth-facilitating tool, its use requires a careful self-exploration on the part of the counselor.

A Practice Exercise for you. See what you would do with the technique of Confrontation-in-action in the following case:

1. You have been seeing James for three months, weekly. You have a good relationship and have done some good work together. James has been dry during your counseling relationship, but yesterday you spoke to his wife who informed you James had hit the bottle again over the weekend. It is Monday afternoon and James comes in for his usual appointment, clean-shaven, sober, but a little shaky.

Counselor: Hi, James. Come on in and sit down. What's going on with you?

Client: Oh, hi. Well, not much. Everything's 'bout the same as usual. I've been doing just fine .... yep, just fine. How's yourself?

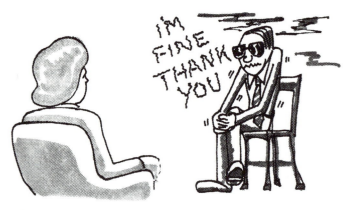

Counselor:

NOTES:

A Practice Exercise for you. See what you would do with the technique of Confrontation-in-action in the following case:

2. You have only seen Mary one time. She has achieved only two weeks sobriety and is leaning very heavily on her counselor and AA to maintain sobriety. She comes in for her second meeting with you two days earlier than her scheduled appointment.

Counselor: Well, Mary, I'm glad to see you, but wasn't really expecting you today. What's up?

Client: Oh, nothing. Nothing at all. I'm feeling **really** fine!! No problems. Just wanted to come by for a little social-type visit. Is that okay?

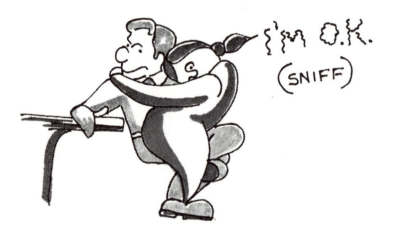

Counselor:

NOTES:

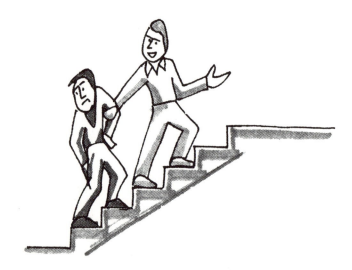

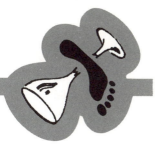

10. POTENCY

Description. This variable is measuring the charismatic or magnetic quality of the counselor. The potent counselor is obviously in command of himself and communicates a dynamic, involved attitude to the client.

Potency-in-action.

Client: (pacing up and down the room, lost in thought) I just want to work harder on that job out there because I **know** things can get done better than they are. I believe I could change a few things for the better, if I just could ....

Counselor: (gets up and starts walking around the room with the client) Golly, Bob, as you were saying that I got a feel for the power and the sensitivity you've got in you! (very expressively) I really **felt** it!!

Client: You really did? You felt **my** power? Well, golly .... (excitedly) You know, I really mean it. I **could** do a lot more out there .... I could ....

Counselor: Go on. You could ....?

Process. Because he is truly involved with his client and doesn't hold back expressing it, the counselor has hooked into the client's potential power bank. This process enables the client to feel his own power and to believe in it. He feels accepted and encouraged to go on and use his potential, as he has just been validated by his counselor as a useful human being. His counselor is also serving as a model for his client—a model of someone who lives effectively with hope and enthusiasm. As the client begins to act from his potential power bank, he will look to his counselor for rewards when he is successful, even in the tiniest way, and for encouragement and understanding when he falters or fails. It is very important that the counselor remembers to praise each small step toward effective living that the client attempts or achieves.

Opposite of Potency-in-action. The counselor who scores low in potency is flat in affect—uninvolved and unexpressive. He is utilizing very little of his own inner power and will consequently be unable to facilitate the discovery or releasing of power in his client. Clients often leave sessions with counselors who lack potency feeling uninspired or depressed. They will often drop out of the counseling relationship, or, if forced to see the counselor, will merely go through the motions.

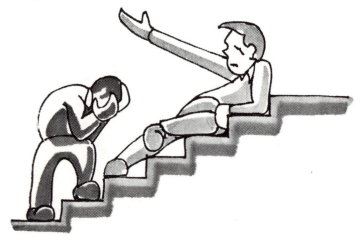

Implications for the alcoholic client. Because of his life history, the alcoholic client feels particularly demoralized and impotent. A counselor who rates high in potency can be a very effective model for the alcoholic client. This stage of modeling after a "potent" counselor may sound too dependent to be healthy, but it is a necessary stage in therapeutic relationship for a client who has had so few good role models. The dependency and "copying behavior" will evolve into a realistic balance of dependence-independence later.

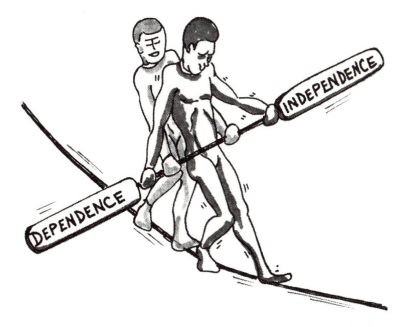

A Practice Exercise for you. Practice a potent response to the client situation described below:

Client: My wife's entire family was over last night. Boy, what a clan. I never felt so mad and confused in all my life. All of 'em talking at once .... never one time ever hearing what anybody else said. They never even noticed I was sober. I kept wanting to tell everybody off, or to tell them what I thought they all sounded like. Sometimes I think maybe I've learned more about livin' than any of 'em. But then ....

Counselor:

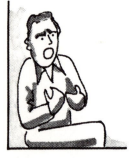

N O T E S :

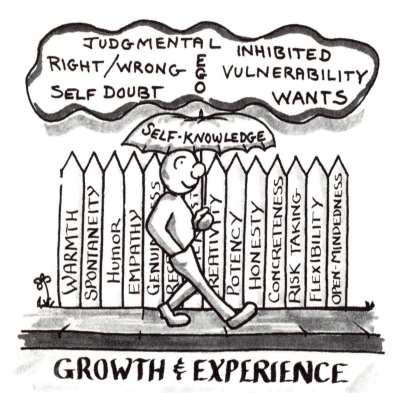

GROWTH & EXPERIENCE

11. SELF-ACTUALIZATION

Description. This variable measures whether or not the counselor is involved in the growth process. A self-actualizing counselor learns from his client while the client is learning from him. He serves as a model of effective, full living. He is able to express himself freely because he does not see himself as "having arrived." He does not have to fall back on roles or phoniness because he is not having to protect himself from becoming known. Because he accepts himself as a finite being with strengths and weaknesses, he does not have to judge or moralize to his clients. He has the capacity for spontaneous warmth and intimacy. He is flexible: if a course of action does not fall into place, he can flow toward other possibilities without becoming incapacitated with anxiety. He feels stress and tension, but he is not immobilized by these feelings. He seeks to know himself more and more, and will risk new behavior in order to grow or discover new truths about himself. He does not lean on dogma or preconceived notions to determine his life, but flows with the "process of becoming," using **his own experiencing** as the test for authenticity. Since he does this for himself, he also trusts and respects others' experiences as valid. He is no longer hung up on what is "right" and "wrong," but looks at the world in a different way. The only "wrong" is when a person blocks getting his needs met so that he operates out of deficiencies in his personal need system; this means that he harms himself and other people in his life in ways that are not clear to anyone involved. "Right" means learning to take care of yourself in a way that satisfies your needs enough that you are free to be a giving person to others.

"Self-actualization" is really a technical word whose definition is based on scientific research. Its chief author is Abraham Maslow. From studies of self-actualizing people, it has been found that when deficiency needs are met, people tend to operate out of "B-needs" (being-needs). B-needs are gratified through love and enhancing one's potentials, and are no longer concerned with ego gratification at the expense of oneself or others. People who rate high on self-actualization scales are more loving and concerned with other people in their society than people who rate low on this scale. Maslow has concluded from this that human nature is basically good, or at least neutral—and that any form of uncovering therapy (learning to understand and accept oneself) releases the basic potential good that is in us, rather than unleashing evil "animal" instincts. He asserts that the selfishness, greed and evil we see in human beings are due to lack of self support or environmental support which causes the individual to operate from deficiency needs.

Self-actualization is not merely a trait or characteristic—it is a description of the whole person in process, encompassing all the other nine personal characteristics which correlate with helping. What does a person do when he self-actualizes? As Maslow humorously asks at one point: "Does he grit his teeth and squeeze?" It might be helpful at this point to describe in behavioral terms some of the things that actually happen when we are in the process of self-actualization.

1. A person will begin experiencing in the moment more fully and vividly, with full concentration and without self-consciousness. Remember when we were adolescents and had the feeling we were always "on stage"—that whatever we were doing, public or private, people (usually "judges") were watching us? In the self-actualization process, this feeling tends to disappear and we begin doing for ourselves, rather than doing for "an audience." This process is tied very closely to the process of creativity— being able to completely unite with the "other" in the moment. The "other" might be a piece of stone if you are a sculptor, or another person if you are a counselor.

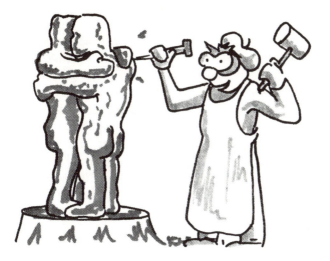

2. The self-actualizer will choose **in the moment** a "growth" choice instead of lying or "weaseling out" when confronted with a painful situation where lying would save him from the confrontation. He begins taking responsibility for his decisions and actions, and experiences a sense of freedom in doing so—though the freedom can sometimes be lonely or painful.

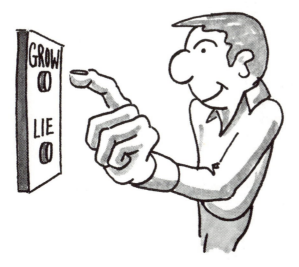

3. A person involved in self-actualizing behavior will begin "checking himself out" to see if an attitude or decision is really **his** feeling or, if it is an unexamined belief system which comes from some significant other in his past, or an idea he picked up from a past revered source. He begins asking himself questions like, "Do I really want to spend all my Sunday afternoons on family picnics, or is this something I am doing because my parents always did it?" He may even discover no one in the family is enjoying this ceremonious event. He begins listening more to his own "impulse voices" and less to the noises of the world.

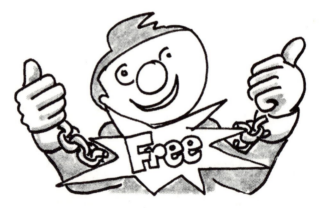

4. A self-actualizing person often will engage in periods of arduous preparation for a chosen task or a newly discovered skill or interest. Quite often, a housewife will go back for a degree. Or a man might change professions in midstream. Values are shifted, life styles become obsolete; some relationships die while others bloom or begin to grow in different directions and deeper dimensions. Sometimes a person considered to be emotionally stable and the rock of his community will enter psychotherapy or behave in ways that seem unpredictable to his closest associates. Often, periods of disorganization and chaos seem to crop up "out of the blue" at the very time in one's life when the pattern has become stabilized and easy.

5. "Peak experiences," (moments of ecstacy, or mystical, religious experiences) can begin occurring to one in the process of self-actualization. These experiences are difficult to describe unless one has experienced them. They are the little moments in life where even the mundane can become sacred. They can occur under a wide variety of circumstances—while being in love, giving birth to a child, listening to music, walking through a busy parking lot, or looking at a sunrise. Besides being just inherently beautiful, these moments can open up new horizons for us, cure a neurosis, give us an insight leading to a new feeling about ourselves, or increase our regard for people or for the world in general. In short, they help to release our fullest potential as human beings.

The self-actualizing counselor is not concerned with teaching in the ordinary sense of the word, but is concerned only with helping the client realize his own way, his own unique style of being in the world. It is the Taoistic attitude—the "non-interfering" way of helping another to unfold, to break through his defenses against himself, to recover himself, or to discover himself.

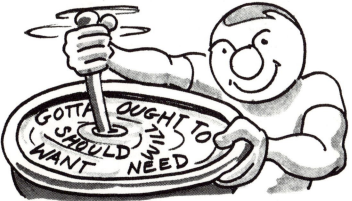

In the self-actualization process, facts and values seem to fuse. This is where a counselor can be so crucial to the process. Let me attempt an explanation, and then an example, of self-actualization counseling in process. People who come for counseling are always in conflict. The conflict is usually centered around the valuing process—"I ought to" versus "I want to," or "I ought to, but I can't."

When we begin examining "ought systems," we discover quickly that there are two kinds of "oughts." There are oughts that are external to us, and there are oughts that are intrinsically locked into our own self system, which when violated produce horrible chaos and confusion internally. Good counseling consists of helping a client discover which oughts are external (really introjects from significant others or from the society at large), and which oughts are actual needs of the client's own organism, which must be listened to and satisfied. If there were indeed such a thing as **complete** self-actualization, what would happen would be that for each of us, **what is** (facts) and **what ought to be** (values) would fuse—our authentic self would fuse with our values, and there would be no more conflict.

Consequently, the self-actualizing counselor must be non-judgmental and concerned with values in a non-moralistic manner, in order to aid his client in the discovery of his own internal and external values, or oughts, and to know the difference between the two.

Self-actualizing counselor in action.

Client: I'm seeing Betty on the side, you know. Sarah doesn't know it. She would **die**!! She's telling everybody we're just about to get married. And you know how much our folks are counting on us marrying. But I'll tell you—Betty is making me feel real good about some things. I feel like I **need** her company .... at least, I just seem to keep going over there a lot .... sort of like a return of the old manhood or something. I don't know. Yeah, that's what it is. She just makes me feel like some kind of MAN! (determined) **I won't** be forced into giving her up just yet!!! I just WON'T!!

Counselor: Sounds like you are choosing a course of action which feels really right to you just now, Bill. I notice, too, though, that this choice doesn't seem all that easy for you to make .... like maybe there's a lot of pain in it for you .... considering the possible reaction

	Sarah and your folks might have if they knew about Betty.
Client:	It's really just awful. I shouldn't be doing this .... boy, am I confused.
Counselor:	I think I know how that dilemma feels, Bill. I have to work on myself a lot about what consequences I'm willing to pay if I choose to do something that I know has a lot of pain in it for someone else. That is sure a tough one alright!!
Client:	Yeah. Well, I **do** know I could lose Sarah either way I go .... I mean, if I don't tell her about Betty and she finds out from someone else, or if I **do** tell her.
Counselor:	What do you get for yourself from your relationship with **Sarah**, Bill? Are you pretty clear on that?

Process. Because the counselor is a searching, growing person himself, he knows life contains ambiguities that do not always have "a correct answer." Note that he is not choosing to relate to his client by lecturing him on the matter of promises and commitments to a fiancée, or living up to his parents' wishes, but is instead accepting the client as a human being who has choices and consequences unique to his own situation. The counselor is also claiming the fact that both he and the client are part of the same human race, with certain needs and dilemmas that are similar. He is enabling his client to reality-test his decision (to continue seeing Betty) against another very real human being (himself). This can lead to clarification of actions and consequences for the client which can, in turn, lead him to face his decision more honestly and directly, based on his **real** internal oughts rather than on appearances or needs which are external to the real human issues involved.

Implications for the alcoholic client. The alcoholic client will grow in relationship with a self-actualizing person, and will begin to actualize himself. He will feel accepted by this kind of counselor in spite of his problems with drinking, which have likely been labeled by his relatives and associates as a moral weakness. He will feel that he has a right to be and that he has a hope for a better life vis-a-vis a self-actualizing person. Dogma, moralizing and preaching will drive the alcoholic to drink every time, more hopeless and discouraged after every moralizing encounter. There is no way a person can be truly self-actualizing and not be a naturally therapeutic individual.

A recovering alcoholic client needs to be supported very carefully in a moral system that he is comfortable with. Even the lowest amount of guilt will often drive him back to the bottle. When your client is sharing with you some moral dilemma he's having, it is crucial that you help him examine his actions very carefully in a completely non-judgmental way. He needs you to help him clarify his behavior and his needs **realistically** within the context of a caring relationship and a climate of human equality.

A Practice Exercise for you. See what response comes naturally for you in relationship with the client described below; and see how your behavior compares with what has been described as "self-actualizing" behavior.

Client: Yep. It's true. I'm flunking out of school and I've really just blown the whole semester—tuition, room and board, and all!! I've really done it this time .... blown every chance I ever had for getting accepted into med school. My dad is going to .... oh, God. I don't know if I can even THINK about going home (puts head in hands, long pause). You know, I never have wanted to be a doctor anyway .... Well, yes I have. I mean, my dad and granddad both are doctors .... oh, brother ....

Counselor:

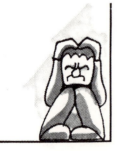

94

NOTES:

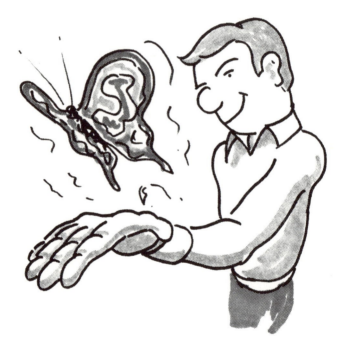

13. A FINAL THOUGHT FOR ALCOHOLISM COUNSELORS

I would like to share with you a simple thought. The alcoholic client needs from you two things:

1. Someone to help him withstand the temptation to drink—because he simply cannot handle alcohol, not one thimbleful;
2. Someone to help him discover his internal oughts and how to realistically meet them—because he cannot survive in the frustration of too many unmet needs.

In short, he must stay away from alcohol and he must develop a good feeling about himself in order to survive.

Many people believe that alcoholism counseling is something unique or mystical, or that it requires a special kind of training and expertise. Many people believe that you cannot counsel with an alcoholic client effectively unless you have experienced alcoholism yourself. Neither belief is true. Alcoholism is a problem in living that affects the **whole person.** For you to be significant in the life of the alcoholic and his family, all you need is your own wholeness—your eyes, your ears, your brain, your heart, and your sensitivity—in other words, your natural ability to be human.

12. GLOSSARY

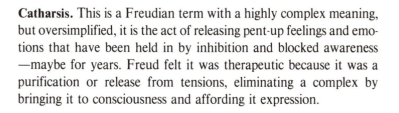

Catharsis. This is a Freudian term with a highly complex meaning, but oversimplified, it is the act of releasing pent-up feelings and emotions that have been held in by inhibition and blocked awareness —maybe for years. Freud felt it was therapeutic because it was a purification or release from tensions, eliminating a complex by bringing it to consciousness and affording it expression.

Corrective Emotional Experience. Quite often a client unconsciously reenacts in his relationship with his counselor, feelings, wishes and experiences involving the client's parents or some other significant figure from his past. In a sense, the client confuses the counselor's identity with the identity of these past figures, usually parents. These held-over feelings from past relationships can be used therapeutically in the present.

For example, if I have a young female client who "transfers" to me feelings she had in relationship with her mother, and her mother made her feel bad about her sexuality, I have the opportunity of correcting my client's emotional experience by making her feel **good** about her sexuality. Since I have become the "mother figure" for the time being, I can replace, or correct, some of this past injustice and can help my client relearn to perceive herself differently. This is called a corrective emotional experience in psychotherapy.

Mirroring. A non-verbal technique of copying exactly what the client is doing behaviorally—hunching his shoulders, scowling, fidgeting, eyes lighting up, etc. This action on the part of the counselor enables the client to see himself in ways he may be unaware of. Since it is very hard to teach our bodies to lie, our non-verbal behavior is usually closer to the truth about our reality than our words.

I was telling a therapist-friend of mine one day that I had decided to take a job I had really talked myself into taking. As I was talking about how glad I was about my decision, she mirrored my non-verbal behavior—frowning, fidgeting, head down, expressionless eyes. I was amazed at how beautifully I had fooled myself into thinking I was glad about my decision. Her mirroring my behavior was more helpful to me than anything she could have said on a rational level. I've never regretted turning down that job!

Morbid Grief. Morbid grief is the technical term for griefwork occurring in unhealthy or indirect ways because of a person's resistance to feeling and expressing **normal** grief at the loss of a loved one. Normal griefwork follows a certain predictable course through various stages—anger, guilt, mourning, acceptance of the loss, and reintegration into a world devoid of the lost person. The amount of time griefwork takes varies with individuals, but usually the process will take somewhere between three months to one year. Morbid, or pathological, grief has several predictable outcomes, too, all of which interfere quite seriously with a person's ability to function and maintain normal relationships with others. Some of the signs of morbid grief are: depersonalization (lack of feeling), agitated depression, flight of ideas, extreme irritability, and some behaviors resembling schizophrenia such as identifying with the lost person (taking on his or her characteristics). When you observe a client with any of these symptoms, it is useful to ask him if someone significant in his life has died, rejected or left him. If so, helping him get on into the avoided feelings will be therapeutic.

Non-judgmental Feedback. My basic assumption as a counselor is that clients deal adequately with their own life problems—**if** they know what they are and can bring all their abilities into action to solve them. The client knows better than I do what decisions are right for him. The art of feeding back to the client what you are experiencing in relation to his personhood, his words, or his actions in a non-judgmental manner is the mark of a good facilitator of personal growth. Non-judgmental feedback is made up of statements which are objective, or "I" statements; they do not contain a "right" or a "wrong" in tone or content.

Example:
Client: I really told her how I felt about it! Was that the right thing to do?
Counselor: You seem very happy with yourself as you talk about having told her off.
Process: The counselor has not "judged" the client's action, but has instead pointed out that the client is acting glad about his action. This feedback is objective, and helps the client see what **he** is really feeling about his own action.

Non-judgmental feedback takes practice, but it is worth every improvement you can possibly make because it keeps you out of the deadly role of "judge," which gives the power and the responsibility to you instead of to the client where it belongs.

Projection. The art of attributing disowned aspects of yourself to others—or, put the other way around—the phenomenon of directly experiencing a feeling as though it were someone else's. If I experience someone else as angry in order to block my awareness of my **own** anger at that person, I am less in touch with the whole transaction and am likely to act or react inappropriately. Projecting and denial go hand in hand: I cannot project onto you a feeling unless I am denying it in myself. The task of the counselor in the face of a client's projection is to help him perceive or experience the feeling as his own.

Reality-Testing. The act of comparing an idea, fantasy, or feeling with one's real experience.

Example:

Client: My sister told me to quit flirting with John so much or he'd get sick of me, so I watch myself around him and try not to come on so strong.

Counselor: How does John act when you flirt with him?

Client: Well, gosh, he seems to love it. He always warms up to me, is more talkative, hugs me a lot, acts really at ease about it.

Counselor: What might be going on in your sister to make her think such a thing about John, I wonder. Sounds more like **her** thing.

Client: You mean my sis may be wrong?

Counselor: Well, which are you going to trust more—your **experience** with John, or your sister's notion of it?

Client: Well, I never .... you know, I never thought of it like that before. (laughs) Old sis .... wonder what her problem is?

Reflecting. A verbal technique of repeating back to the client the essence of what he said. "You say you are happy at home but you don't particularly like weekends?" Often something will clarify for a client when he hears his very own words coming back to him. Many times the things we say are contradictory or have several meanings on several levels, and we just have never taken the time to discover what it all means to us. This is a very common way we all keep ourselves confused. The art of reflecting can slow a person down and cause him to examine more closely the assumptions that underlie his thoughts and actions.

Stuck. This is a Gestalt therapy term, coined by Fritz Perls, meaning this: If I am working with a client along a certain line of blocked awareness and he resists or balks, either trying to put the responsibility on me to do his "work," or telling me that I am really not in tune with where he is, I may get lost and become blocked myself, truly not knowing where to go next, or not willing to go in the direction the client is trying to lead **me**. At a time like this, I am stuck and the most productive act I can make is to claim this openly to my client. "I am stuck right now and cannot think of a way to go with you." This declaration always produces some action on the part of the client. Often it will add to his reasons for resisting you. Whatever it produces (I've even had a dialogue with **myself** at a time like this: "Jacquie, you are stuck right now, what in the world do you suppose is going on here?," etc.) will be material to work with and will move the session out of a bottleneck. This honest action on your part shows the client you are human. It also puts the responsibility on him to work. Trying to fake it when you are honestly stuck **never** works. You will either increase the client's resistance, or you will waste both his time and yours in inauthentic activity.

Unconscious Denial. A psychological defense mechanism which serves the purpose of keeping unacceptable material on an unconscious (unaware) level so that it is not available to the personality for reality-testing. By "unacceptable material" I mean anything about yourself or your world that does not fit in with the psychological system you are consciously using for survival, or anything that would make you feel too guilty or ashamed to handle without some personality disintegration.

Unfinished Business. Perhaps the major consequence of blocked awareness is the phenomenon of unfinished business. Need cycles cannot become completed, tension is aroused but not reduced, and affect mounts but is unexpressed. Little new can happen in the ensuing constriction and frustration when a person is experiencing an overwhelming amount of unfinished business. These unresolved emotional needs carry over into my present relationship with my client, distorting and distracting my ability to listen and involve fully with him. Unfinished business can go a long way back into my past, such as matters pertaining to my relationship with authority figures due to unresolved conflicts with my father—or it can be a very recent piece of unfinished business left unresolved just before I entered the room. Clients can sense when you are not truly "with" them, anyway, so I have found it better to openly claim what is going on with me to my client (he is usually imagining something worse!): "Listen, Bob, I just had a very unpleasant experience with one of my bosses and my feelings are still raw. Let's have a cup of coffee and just chit-chat a minute while I take time to settle down."

When you are aware that some of your unfinished business really cannot be resolved quickly, just being aware of it helps. Here is an example of a counselor's way of handling his own need to be authentic when he is aware of an area of unfinished business in him that dates a long way back: "John, as you begin talking about your problems with your dad, I am aware that I've still got some pretty bad feelings about my own father I haven't worked out yet. I want to be sure I don't get my needs mixed up with yours. I'll need to check us both out very carefully as we go into this. You stop me if I get too far off in trying to hear your problem, okay?"

References

The chief investigators responsible for these counselor variable studies are the following:

Berenson, B.G., Mitchell, J.M. and Laney, R.C., "Level of Therapist Functioning, Types of Confrontation and Type of Patient." *Journal of Clinical Psychology,* 1969, 25, 111-113.

Bergen, A.E., "Some Implications of Psychotherapy Research for Therapeutic Practice." *Journal of Abnormal Psychology,* 1966, 4, 235-246.

Cannon, J.R. and Carkhuff, R.R., "Effects of Rater Level of Functioning and Experience Upon the Discrimination of Facilitative Conditions." *Journal of Consulting and Clinical Psychology,* 1969, 32, 189-194.

——————— "Helping and Human Relations: A Primer for Lay and Professional Helpers." *Selection and Training,* Vol 1. New York: Holt, Rinehart and Winston, Inc., 1969.

Carkhuff, R.R. and Berenson, B.G., *Beyond Counseling and Therapy.* New York: Holt, Rinehart and Winston, Inc., 1967.

Collingwood, T.R. and Renz, L. "The Effects of Client Confrontations upon Levels of Immediacy Offered by High and Low Functioning Counselors." *Journal of Clinical Psychology,* 1969, 25, 224-226.

Foulds, M.L., "Self Actualization and the Communication of Facilitative Conditions during Counselling." *Journal of Counselling Psychology,* 1969, 16, 132-136.

Truax, C.B. and Carkhuff, R.R., *Toward Effective Counselling and Psychotherapy: Training and Practice.* Chicago: Aldine Publishing Company, 1967.

Wolf, S. "An Investigation of Counsellor Type, Client Type, Level of Facilitative Conditions and Client Outcome." (Doctoral Dissertation, The Catholic University of America), *Dissertation Abstracts International,* 1970, 31, Order No. 70-22,093.

Wolf, S. "Counseling: For Better or Worse." *ADPA, Selected Papers,* 23rd Annual Meeting, September 10-15, 1972, Atlanta, Georgia.

Note: Dr. Wolf is credited with pulling together the above research findings on counselor effectiveness. They also correlate with the findings of Carl Rogers and Abraham Maslow in their studies of the therapeutic encounter and self-actualizing behavior.

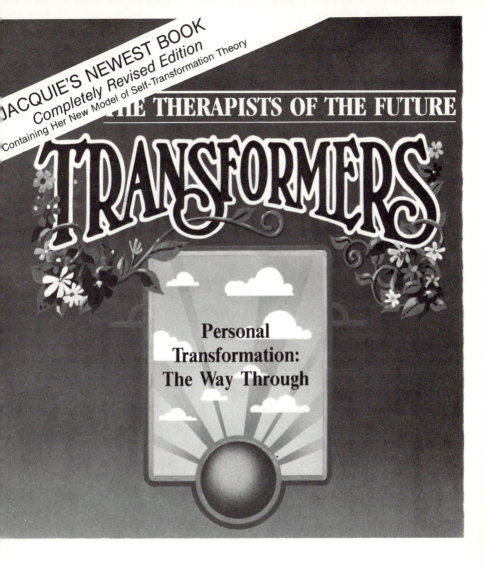

JACQUIE'S NEWEST BOOK

Completely Revised Edition

Containing Her New Model of Self-Transformation Theory

THE THERAPISTS OF THE FUTURE

TRANSFORMERS

Personal Transformation: The Way Through

From the book . . .

"Transformers work with what *is* about us, not what 'ought to be' by someone else's standards. And by their positive acceptance of us — their total endorsement of our being — they serve as catalysts for lifting us to our highest, most integrated level. They work from above, downward — from the perspective of perfection, they weed out the *im*perfection, focusing on clearing the way for more and more of the authentic masterpiece to shine through."

Distributed by The Eupsychian Press, P.O. Box 3090, Austin, Texas 78764.

$11.95 + $1.50 postage for the first copy, $.50 postage each additional copy.

Texas residents add 8% sales tax.